THE COMPL___ _ ___

DIET COOKBOOK:

Easy and Healthy Recipes for People Who Care About Their Health.

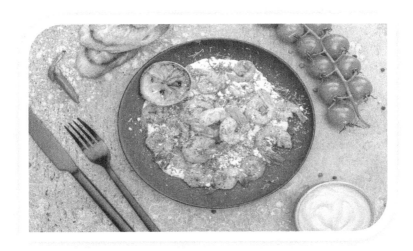

Samuel Hayes

TABLE OF CONTENTS

INTRODUCTION

The "dash diet" refers to dietary methods for lowering blood pressure. This book is about a specialized diet for those with high blood pressure. Even if you've had high blood pressure for some time, this book is a great resource for you. It is well-known that lifestyle and dietary habits can have a greater impact on your health than medication. You'll find a recipe for just about anything in this book.

In this book, you'll find DASH diet dishes that are simple to follow and can be produced in no time. The DASH diet has witnessed a dramatic rise in popularity over the past decade. In recent years, more and more people have become aware of the Dietary Approaches to Stop Hypertension diet's ability to reduce high blood pressure. The DASH diet emphasizes foods high in potassium, calcium, and magnesium while minimizing sodium consumption. In addition, processed carbs, fizzy beverages, and sugar are discouraged in the diet.

As a result of today's hectic lifestyle, many people find themselves fatigued and tempted to overeat. People in their 30s are now experiencing heart problems that were previously only observed in the elderly. This has increased the urgency of finding ways to return to a healthy lifestyle. As a result, a growing number of people are considering the DASH diet as a means of reducing such diseases. High blood pressure can be combated with the help of this cookbook, which is prepared in an easy-to-follow manner for both experts and novices. Every meal of the day is covered here, from breakfast to dinner.

People who are trying to manage their blood pressure tend to eat plain, unappetizing foods. The majority of us give up on such a regimen when we don't have a taste for it. The recipes in this cookbook are designed to help you eat a wider variety of foods in an effort to improve your health. In addition to assisting you to control your blood sugar, these DASH diet recipes will also allow you to have fun with the cooking process.

Keeping your sodium intake under control might be beneficial. Other than salt, the DASH diet requires people to consume a large amount of fruit and vegetables. Fiber and vitamins in fruits and vegetables help to keep blood pressure and cholesterol levels in check and aid in reducing them. When following the DASH diet, it's best to avoid eating a lot of red meat, but if you must, opt for seafood and chicken instead. This book has a section devoted to sweets.

CHAPTER 1 DASH DIET TIPS

The National Heart, Lung, and Blood Institute (NHLBI) is promoting the DASH diet, which stands for dietary approaches to prevent hypertension, to do just that: prevent hypertension. It focuses on foods high in potassium, calcium, protein, and fiber that lower blood pressure, such as whole grains, fruits, vegetables, lean protein, and low-fat dairy. Sugar-sweetened beverages and sweets are likewise discouraged by DASH, as are fatty meats, full-fat dairy products, and tropical oils high in saturated fat. Capping your salt intake at 2,300 milligrams a day is also part of the DASH diet, which you will eventually lower to 1,500 mg. The DASH diet is well-balanced and can be maintained for an extended period of time. StatPearls, the world's best source of medical information, shows that the DASH diet is linked to a lower risk of cardiovascular disease.

DASH diet tips:

1. You should include a serving of vegetables to your lunch and dinner.

2. When eating or snacking, include a piece of fruit in your diet. If you're going to utilize dried or canned fruit, make sure there isn't any sugar added to them.

3. Cut back on the amount of margarine, butter, or salad dressing you typically use, and swap in fat-free or low-fat condiments instead.

4. Low-fat or skim dairy products can be consumed in the same way as full-fat or cream-based dairy products.

5. Limit yourself to six ounces of beef a day. Make a few of your meals meatless.

6. Increasing your intake of vegetables and dry beans is a smart idea.

7. If you don't want potato chips or sweets, try almonds that aren't salted, fruit, low-fat and fat-free yogurt,

frozen yogurt, and popcorn that isn't flavored or butter-flavored.

8. Reduce sodium intake by reading the nutrition facts on food labels.

9. Use spices or flavorings that are sodium-free in place of salt.

10. When cooking rice, pasta, or hot porridge, avoid adding salt.

11. Choose fresh, frozen, or canned veggies in their natural state

12. Choose skinless poultry, fish, and lean cuts of meat that are fresh or frozen.

13. Read food labels and select salt-free or low-sodium options.

Chapter 2
Breakfast

CREAMY APPLE-AVOCADO SMOOTHIE

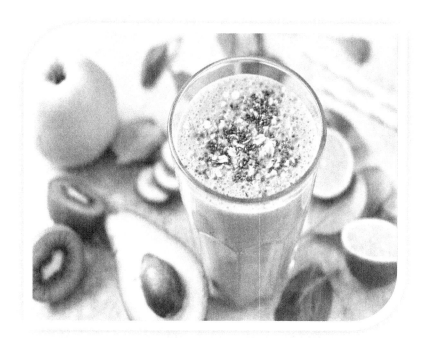

| Prep time: 15 minutes | Cook time: 15 minutes | Servings: 2 |

Ingredients

- Medium avocado - 1/2, peeled and pitted
- Medium apple - 1, chopped
- Baby spinach leaves - 1 cup
- Nonfat vanilla Greek yogurt - 1 cup
- Water - 1/2 to 1 cup
- Ice - 1 cup
- Freshly squeezed lemon juice (optional)

6

Method

1. Blend all the ingredients in a blender, except for the lemon juice.
2. Add lemon juice and serve.

Nutritional Facts Per Serving

- Calories: 200
- Fat: 7g
- Carb: 27g
- Protein: 10g
- Sodium: 56mg

STRAWBERRY, ORANGE, AND BEET SMOOTHIE

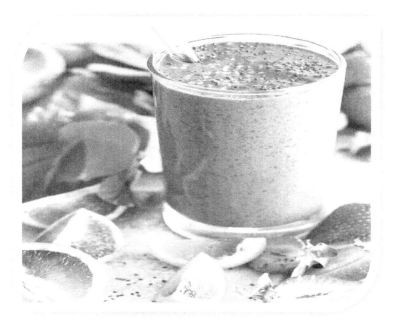

| Prep time: 5 minutes | Cook time: 20 minutes | Servings: 2 |

Ingredients

- Nonfat milk - 1 cup
- Frozen strawberries - 1 cup
- Medium beet - 1, cooked, peeled, and cubed
- Orange - 1, peeled and quartered
- Frozen banana - 1, peeled and chopped
- Nonfat vanilla Greek yogurt - 1 cup
- Ice 1 cup

Method

1. Blend everything in a blender and serve.

Nutritional Facts Per Serving

- Calories: 266
- Fat: 0g
- Carb: 51g
- Protein: 15g
- Sodium: 104mg

BLUEBERRY-VANILLA YOGURT SMOOTHIE

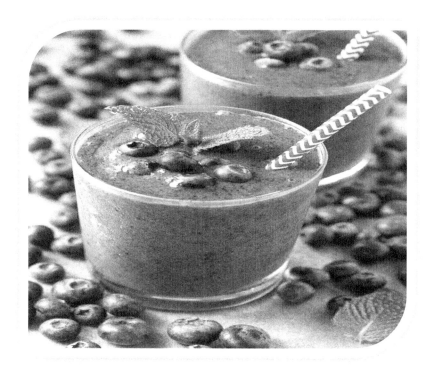

| Prep time: 5 minutes | Cook time: 5 minutes | Servings: 2 |

Ingredients

- Frozen blueberries - 1 1/2 cups
- Nonfat vanilla Greek yogurt - 1 cup
- Frozen banana - 1, peeled and sliced
- Nonfat or low-fat milk - 1/2 cup
- Ice - 1 cup

Method

1. In a blender, blend everything until smooth. Serve.

Nutritional Facts Per Serving

- Calories: 228
- Fat: 1g
- Carb: 45g
- Protein: 12g
- Sodium: 63mg

GREEK YOGURT OAT PANCAKES

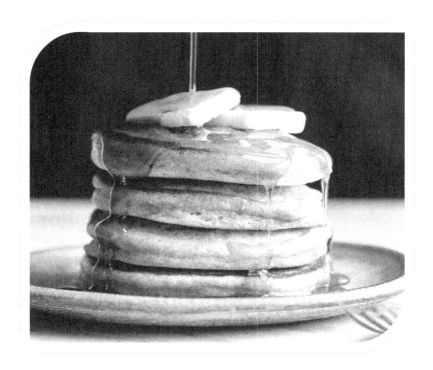

Prep time: 15 minutes	Cook time: 10 to 15 minutes	Servings: 2

Ingredients

- Egg whites - 6
- Rolled oats - 1 cup
- Plain nonfat Greek yogurt - 1 cup
- Medium banana - 1, peeled and sliced
- Ground cinnamon - 1 teaspoon
- Baking powder - 1 teaspoon

Method

1. Blend everything in a blender. Grease a skillet with cooking spray.

2. Put 1/3 cup batter onto the griddle and cook for 5 minutes. Flip and cook for 2 minutes more or until golden.

3. Repeat with the remaining batter and serve.

Nutritional Facts Per Serving

- Calories: 318
- Fat: 4g
- Carb: 47g
- Protein: 28g
- Sodium: 467mg

STUFFED BREAKFAST PEPPERS

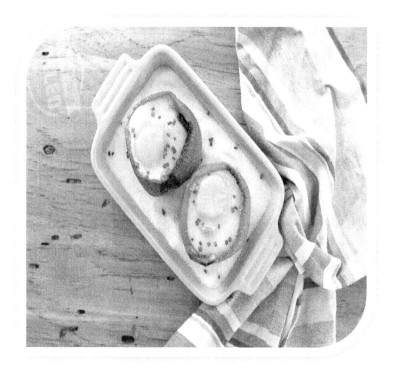

| Prep time: 15 minutes | Cook time: 45 minutes | Servings: 4 |

Ingredients

- Bell peppers - 4 (any color)
- Frozen spinach - 1 (16-oz.) bag
- Eggs - 4
- Shredded low-fat cheese - 1/4 cup (optional)
- Freshly ground black pepper

Method

1. Preheat the oven to 400 F. Aluminum foil should be used to line a baking dish. Remove the pepper's tops and discard the seeds. Remove the tops and seeds.

2. Bake the peppers in the baking dish for approximately 15 minutes. While the peppers bake, defrost the spinach and drain any excess moisture. Remove the peppers and fill the bottoms with the defrosted spinach equally.

3. Crack an egg inside each pepper and place it on top of the spinach. Each egg should be topped with a spoonful of cheddar (if used) and seasoned with freshly ground black pepper to taste.

4. Bake for 15–20 minutes.

Nutritional Facts Per Serving

- Calories: 136
- Fat: 5g
- Carb: 15g
- Protein: 11g
- Sodium: 131mg

APPLE-APRICOT BROWN RICE BREAKFAST PORRIDGE

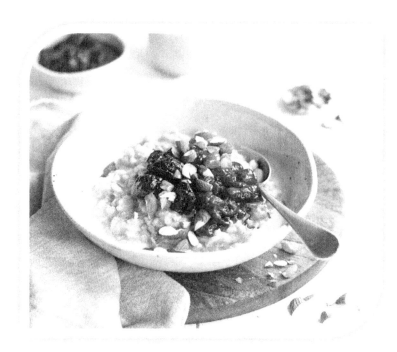

| Prep time: 15 minutes | Cook time: 8 minutes | Servings: 4 |

Ingredients

- Cooked brown rice - 3 cups
- Nonfat or low-fat milk - ¼ cups
- Lightly packed brown sugar - 2 tablespoons
- Dried apricots - 4, chopped
- Medium apple - 1, cored and diced
- Ground cinnamon - 3/4 teaspoon
- Vanilla extract - 3/4 teaspoon

16

Method

1. Combine the rice, cinnamon, apple, apricots, sugar, milk in a saucepan.

2. Boil on medium heat. Then cook for 2 to 3 minutes on low heat.

3. Turn off the heat and add the vanilla extract. Serve.

Nutritional Facts Per Serving

- Calories: 260
- Fat: 2g
- Carb: 57g
- Protein: 7g
- Sodium: 50mg

EGG WHITE BREAKFAST MIX

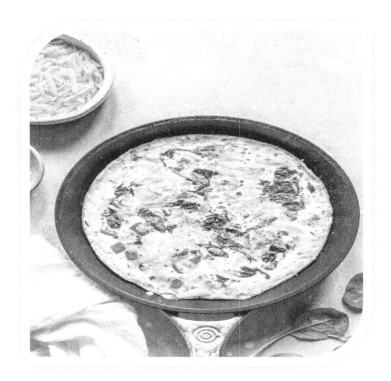

| Prep time: 10 minutes | Cook time: 10 minutes | Servings: 4 |

Ingredients

- Yellow onion - 1, chopped
- Plum tomatoes - 3, chopped
- Spinach - 10 oz., chopped
- Pinch black pepper
- Water - 2 tablespoons
- Egg whites - 12
- Cooking spray

Method

1. Mix the egg whites with water and pepper in a bowl. Grease a pan with cooking spray. Add ¼ of the egg whites, spread into the pan, and cook for 2 minutes.

2. Spoon ¼ of the spinach, onion, tomatoes, and fold to a plate. Serve.

Nutritional Facts Per Serving

- Calories: 31
- Fat: 2g
- Carb: 0g
- Protein: 3g
- Sodium: 55mg

PESTO OMELET

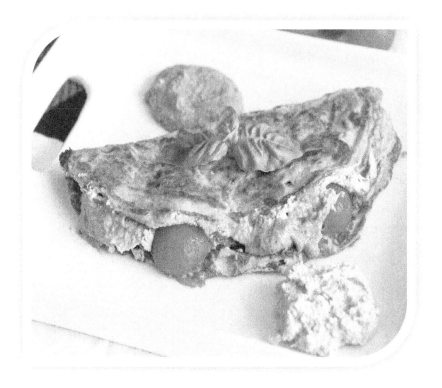

| Prep time: 10 minutes | Cook time: 6 minutes | Servings: 2 |

Ingredients

- Olive oil - 2 teaspoons
- Handful cherry tomatoes, chopped
- Pistachio pesto - 3 tablespoons
- Pinch black pepper
- Eggs - 4

Method

1. In a bowl, combine the cherry tomatoes, eggs, black pepper, and pistachio pesto and mix well.

2. Add the eggs, mix, and spread into the pan. Cook for 3 minutes. Flip and cook for 3 minutes more. Serve.

Nutritional Facts Per Serving

- Calories: 240
- Fat: 9g
- Carb: 23g
- Protein: 17g
- Sodium: 292mg

QUINOA BOWLS

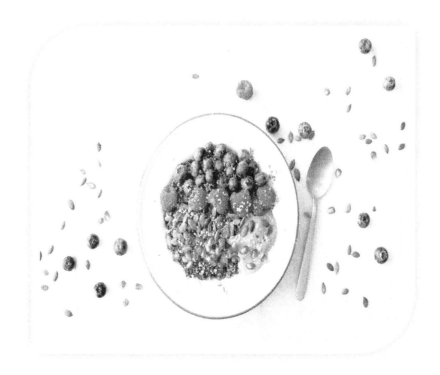

| Prep time: 10 minutes | Cook time: 20 minutes | Servings: 2 |

Ingredients

- Peach - 1, sliced
- Quinoa - 1/3 cup, rinsed
- Low-fat milk - 2/3 cup
- Vanilla extract - 1/2 teaspoon
- Brown sugar - 2 teaspoons
- Raspberries - 12
- Blueberries - 14

Method

1. Mix the milk, sugar, quinoa, and vanilla in a pan. Simmer over medium heat. Cover the pan. Cook for 20 minutes and flip.

2. Divide this mix into two bowls. Top each with raspberries and blueberries and serve.

Nutritional Facts Per Serving

- Calories: 170
- Fat: 3g
- Carb: 31g
- Protein: 6g
- Sodium: 120mg

STRAWBERRY SANDWICH

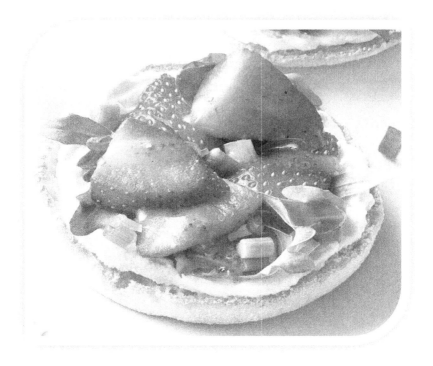

| Prep time: 10 minutes | Cook time: 5 minutes | Servings: 4 |

Ingredients

- Low-fat cream cheese - 8 oz., soft
- Stevia - 1 tablespoon
- Lemon zest - 1 teaspoon, grated
- Whole-wheat English muffins - 4, toasted
- Strawberries - 2 cups, sliced

Method

1. In a food processor, add the stevia, cream cheese, and lemon zest and blend well.

2. Spread 1 tbsp of this mix on one muffin half and top with some of the sliced strawberries.

3. Repeat with the rest of the muffin halves and serve.

Nutritional Facts Per Serving

- Calories: 150
- Fat: 7g
- Carb: 23g
- Protein: 2g
- Sodium: 70mg

APPLE QUINOA MUFFINS

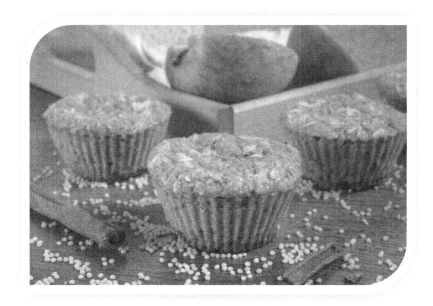

| Prep time: 10 minutes | Cook time: 35 minutes | Servings: 4 |

Ingredients

- Natural unsweetened applesauce - 1/2 cup
- Banana - 1 cup, peeled and mashed
- Quinoa - 1 cup
- Old-fashioned oats - 2 and 1/2 cups
- Almond milk - 1/2 cup
- Stevia - 2 tablespoons
- Vanilla extract - 1 teaspoon
- Water - 1 cup
- Cooking spray

- Cinnamon powder - 1 teaspoon
- Apple - 1, cored, peeled, and chopped

Method

1. Put the water in a pan. Bring to a simmer and add quinoa. Cook for 15 minutes. Fluff and transfer to a bowl.
2. Add all ingredients and stir.
3. Divide into a muffin pan greased with cooking spray.
4. Preheat oven to 375 F and bake for 20 minutes.
5. Serve.

Nutritional Facts Per Serving

1. Calories: 241
2. Fat: 11g
3. Carb: 31g
4. Protein: 5g
5. Sodium: 251mg

VERY BERRY MUESLI

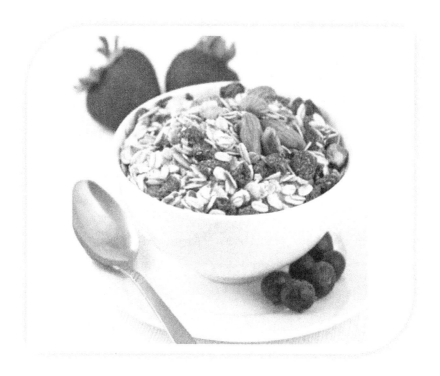

| Prep time: 15 minutes | Cook time: 10 minutes | Servings: 2 |

Ingredients

- Oats - 1 cup
- Fruit-flavored yogurt - 1 cup
- Milk - 1/2 cup
- Salt - 1/8 teaspoon
- Dried Raisins -1/2 cup
- Chopped apple - 1/2 cup
- Frozen blueberries - 1/2 cup

- Chopped walnuts - 1/4 cup

Method

1. Combine oats, yogurt, and salt in a bowl. Mix well and cover tightly.
2. Fridge overnight.
3. Add your raisins and apples and fold.
4. Top with walnuts and serve.

Nutritional Facts Per Serving

- Calories: 195
- Fat: 4g
- Carb: 31g
- Protein: 6g
- Sodium: 0mg

BACON BITS

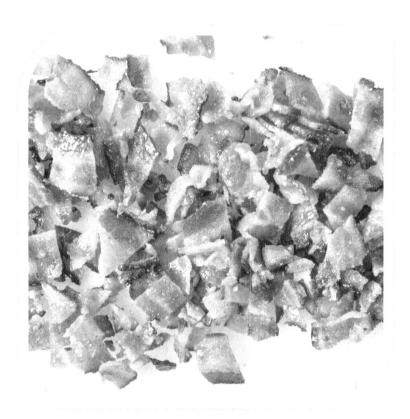

| Prep time: 15 minutes | Cook time: 60 minutes | Servings: 4 |

Ingredients

- Millet 1 cup
- Water 5 cups
- Diced sweet potato 1 cup
- Ground cinnamon 1 teaspoon
- Brown sugar 2 tablespoons

- Medium diced apple 1
- Honey 1/4 cup

Method

1. In a large saucepan, combine the sugar, sweet potato, cinnamon, water, and millet. Stir everything together, then bring it to a boil over high heat.

2. Reduce the heat to a low simmer. Continue cooking in this manner for approximately an hour, or until the water is completely absorbed and the millet is cooked.

3. Combine the remaining ingredients in a bowl and serve.

Nutritional Facts Per Serving

- Calories: 136
- Fat: 1g
- Carb: 28.5g
- Protein: 3.1g
- Sodium: 120mg

TURKEY SAUSAGE AND MUSHROOM STRATA

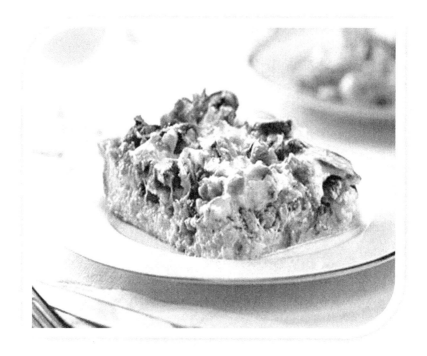

Prep time: 15 minutes	Cook time: 20 to 30 minutes	Servings: 12

Ingredients

- Cubed ciabatta bread - 8 oz.
- Chopped turkey sausage -12 oz.
- Milk - 2 cups
- Shredded cheddar - 4 oz.
- Large egg - 3
- Egg substitute - 12 oz.

32

- Chopped green onion - 1/2 cup
- Diced mushroom - 1 cup
- Paprika - 1/2 teaspoon
- Pepper - 1/2 teaspoon
- Grated parmesan cheese - 2 tablespoons

Method

1. Preheat the oven to 400F. Arrange the bread cubes flat on a baking pan and toast for approximately 8 minutes. Cook the sausage, occasionally stirring, until fully browned and crumbles.
2. In a bowl, combine salt, pepper, paprika, parmesan cheese, egg substitute, eggs, cheddar cheese, and milk. Add the rest of the fixings and mix.
3. Place the mixture in a baking dish, cover tightly, and place in the refrigerator overnight.
4. Remove the cover from the dish. Bake at 350F until golden brown.
5. Cut into slices to serve.

Nutritional Facts Per Serving

- Calories: 288.2
- Fat: 12.4g
- Carb: 18.2g
- Protein: 24.3g
- Sodium: 355mg

CARROT CAKE OVERNIGHT OATS

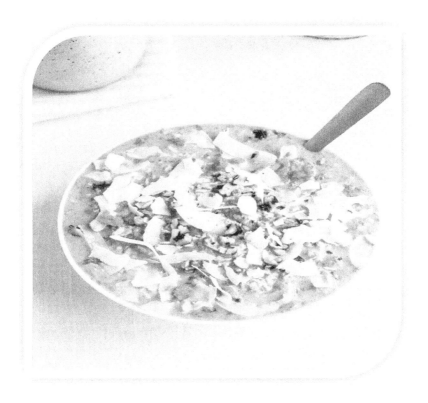

| Prep time: Overnight | Cook time: 2 minutes | Servings: 1 |

Ingredients

- Rolled oats - 1/2 cup
- Plain nonfat or low-fat Greek yogurt - 1/2 cup
- Nonfat or low-fat milk - 1/2 cup
- Shredded carrot - 1/4 cup
- Raisins - 2 tablespoons
- Ground cinnamon - 1/2 teaspoon

- Chopped walnuts (optional) - 1 to 2 tablespoons

Method

1. Mix all the ingredients in a jar. Cover and shake well. Refrigerate overnight.
2. Serve.

Nutritional Facts Per Serving

- Calories: 331
- Fat: 3g
- Carb: 59g
- Protein: 22g
- Sodium: 141mg

MEDITERRANEAN TOAST

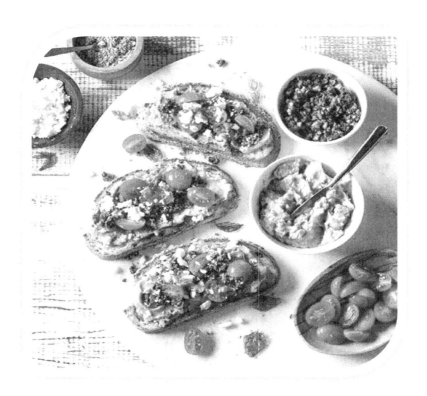

| Prep time: 10 minutes | Cook time: 0 minutes | Servings: 2 |

Ingredients

- Reduced-fat crumbled feta - 1 1/2 teaspoon
- Sliced Greek olives - 3
- Mashed avocado - 1/4
- Whole wheat bread - 1 slice
- Roasted red pepper hummus - 1 tablespoon
- Sliced cherry tomatoes - 3
- Sliced hardboiled egg - 1

Method

1. Toast the bread and top it with ¼ mashed avocado and 1 tbsp. hummus.
2. Add the cherry tomatoes, olives, hardboiled egg, and feta. Season and serve.

Nutritional Facts Per Serving

- Calories: 333.7
- Fat: 17g
- Carb: 33.3g
- Protein: 16.3g
- Sodium: 19mg

MUSHROOM FRITTATA

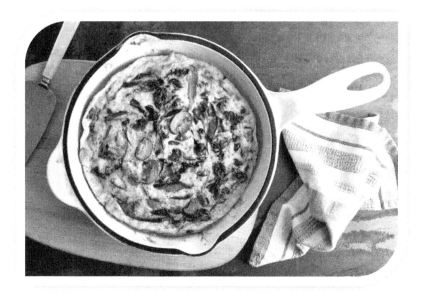

| Prep time: 10 minutes | Cook time: 10 minutes | Servings: 2 |

Ingredients

- Unsalted butter- 1 tsp, melted
- Large brown mushroom - 1, sliced
- Chopped oyster mushroom - ½ cup
- Minced onion - 2 tbsp.
- Eggs - 3 large
- Sour cream - ½ cup
- Black pepper to taste
- Cherry tomatoes to serve
- Basil to serve

Method

1. Melt the butter in a saucepan and gently cook the onion and mushrooms for 3–4 minutes.

2. Whisk together the eggs and sour cream. Season with freshly ground black pepper.

3. Preheat your oven's grill function.

4. Add the egg mixture and cook on low heat for 2 minutes.

5. Place the pan on the grill for about 1-2 minutes, or until the frittata's top is a gorgeous golden hue.

6. Arrange cherry tomatoes and basil in the center of the frittata. Cut and serve while still warm.

Nutritional Facts Per Serving

- Calories: 232
- Fat: 15g
- Carb: 7g
- Protein: 18g
- Sodium: 329mg

FRUITY BREAKFAST MUFFINS

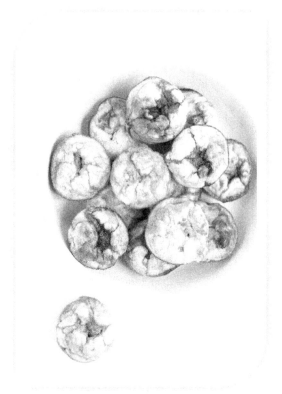

| Prep time: 15 minutes | Cook time: 22 minutes | Servings: 6 |

Ingredients

- Cake flour - 1 cup
- Rolled oats - ½ cup
- Baking powder - 1 tsp
- Mixed spice - ½ tsp
- Ripe bananas - 2
- Castor sugar - 1/3 cup

- Vanilla essence - ½ tsp
- Sunflower oil - ¼ cup
- Egg - 1
- Fresh cranberries - 1 cup

Method

1. Preheat the oven to 350OF.
2. In a mixing bowl, sift together the cake flour, baking powder, and mixed spices. Then stir in the oats.
3. Mash the bananas in a separate bowl and add the caster sugar. Combine thoroughly, then whisk in the vanilla, oil, and egg.
4. In a bowl, mix together the dry and wet ingredients, then add the cranberries.
5. Spray and cook a 6-cup muffin tray, then divide the mixture evenly between the muffin cups.
6. Cook for 20 to 22 minutes.

Nutritional Facts Per Serving

- Calories: 305
- Fat: 11g
- Carb: 47g
- Protein: 7g
- Sodium: 66mg

Chapter 3
Lunch

ARTICHOKE AND SPINACH CHICKEN

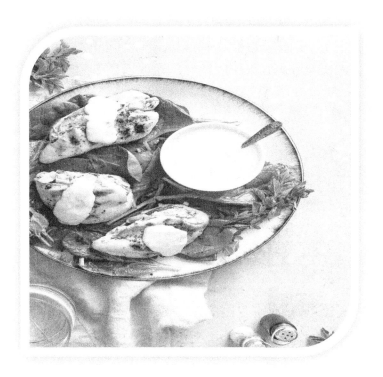

| Prep time: 15 minutes | Cook time: 5 minutes | Servings: 4 |

Ingredients

- Baby spinach - 10 oz.

- Crushed red pepper flakes - 1/2 teaspoon

- Chopped artichoke hearts -14 oz.

- No-salt-added tomato sauce - 28 oz.

- Olive oil - 2 tablespoons

- Boneless and skinless chicken breasts - 4

Method

1. Heat a pan with oil. Add chicken and red pepper flakes and cook for 5 minutes.

2. Add tomato sauce, artichokes, spinach, and toss. Cook for 10 minutes. Serve.

Nutritional Facts Per Serving

- Calories: 212
- Fat: 3g
- Carb: 16g
- Protein: 20g
- Sodium: 418mg

PUMPKIN AND BLACK BEANS CHICKEN

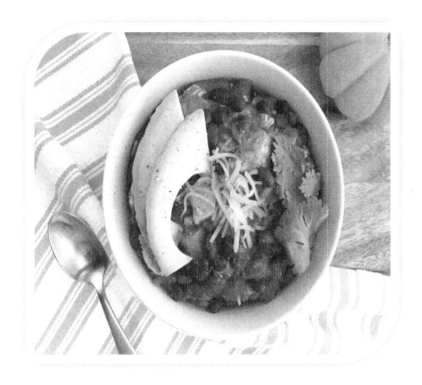

| Prep time: 15 minutes | Cook time: 25 minutes | Servings: 4 |

Ingredients

- Olive oil - 1 tablespoon
- Chopped cilantro - 1 tablespoon
- Coconut milk - 1 cup
- Canned black beans - 15 oz., drained
- Skinless and boneless chicken breasts - 1 pound
- Water - 1 cup
- Pumpkin flesh 1/2 cup

Method

1. Heat a pan with oil. Add chicken and cook for 5 minutes. Add the black beans, pumpkin, milk, and water. Cover and cook for 20 minutes.

2. Add cilantro and serve.

Nutritional Facts Per Serving

- Calories: 254
- Fat: 6g
- Carb: 16g
- Protein: 22g
- Sodium: 92mg

MEDITERRANEAN TURKEY BREAST

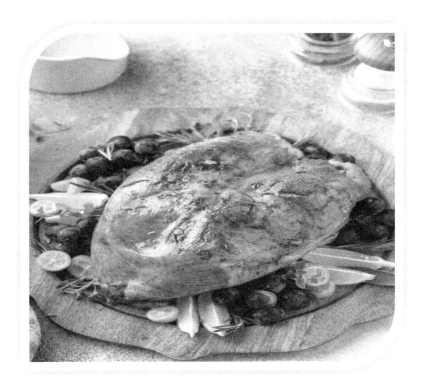

| Prep time: 15 minutes | Cook time: 35 minutes | Servings: 6 |

Ingredients

- Turkey breast - 4 pounds
- Flour - 3 tablespoons
- Chicken stock - 3/4 cup
- Garlic cloves - 4, chopped
- Dried oregano - 1 teaspoon
- Fresh lemon juice - ½ of lemon
- Sun-dried tomatoes - 1/2 cup, chopped

- Olives - 1/2 cup, chopped
- Onion - 1, chopped
- Pepper - 1/4 teaspoon
- Salt - 1/2 teaspoon

Method

1. Add the salt, pepper, onion, olives, tomatoes, lemon juice, oregano, garlic, and turkey breast to a slow cooker.
2. Add half stock and cook for 4 hours.
3. Whisk remaining stock and flour in a bowl and add to the slow cooker
4. Cover and cook for 30 minutes more. Serve.

Nutritional Facts Per Serving

- Calories: 537
- Fat: 9.7g
- Carb: 29.6g
- Protein: 79.1g
- Sodium: 330mg

FAJITA PORK STRIPS

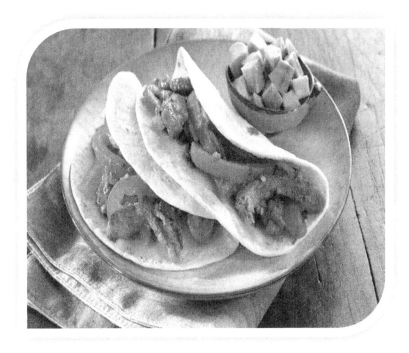

| Prep time: 10 minutes | Cook time: 35 minutes | Servings: 2 |

Ingredients

- Pork sirloin - 16 oz.
- Fajita seasonings - 1 tablespoon
- Canola oil - 1 tablespoon

Method

1. Cut the pork sirloin into the strips and sprinkle with fajita seasonings and canola oil.
2. Then transfer the meat to the baking tray in one layer.

3. Bake it for 35 minutes at 365F. Stir the meat every 10 minutes. Serve.

Nutritional Facts Per Serving

- Calories: 184
- Fat: 0g
- Carb: 1.3g
- Protein: 18.5g
- Sodium: 157mg

TOMATO BEEF

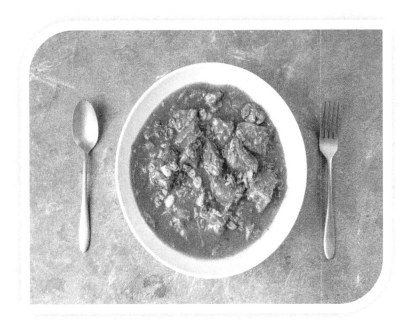

| Prep time: 10 minutes | Cook time: 17 minutes | Servings: 2 |

Ingredients

- Chuck shoulder steaks - 2
- Tomato sauce - 1/4 cup
- Olive oil - 1 tablespoon

Method

1. Preheat the grill to 390F. Brush the steaks with tomato sauce and olive oil.

2. Grill the meat for 9 minutes.

3. Then flip it on another side and cook for 8 minutes more.

51

Nutritional Facts Per Serving

- Calories: 247
- Fat: 17.1g
- Carb: 1.7g
- Protein: 21.4g
- Sodium: 231mg

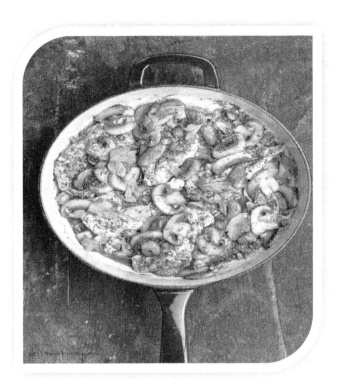

Prep time: 15 minutes	Cook time: 6 hours & 10 minutes	Servings: 2

Ingredients

- Chicken breasts - 2, skinless and boneless
- Mushrooms - 1 cup, sliced
- Onion - 1, sliced
- Chicken stock - 1 cup
- Thyme - 1/2 teaspoon, dried
- Pepper & salt to taste

Method

1. Add everything to the slow cooker.
2. Cook on low for 6 hours. Serve.

Nutritional Facts Per Serving

- Calories: 313
- Fat: 11.3g
- Carb: 6.9g
- Protein: 44.3g
- Sodium: 541mg

FRUIT SHRIMP SOUP

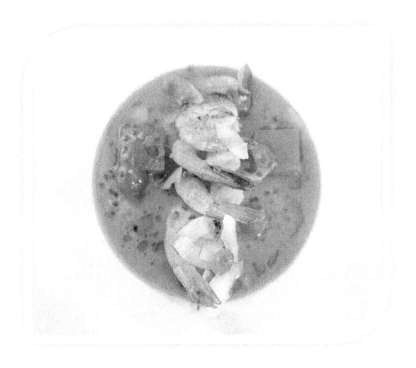

| Prep time: 10 minutes | Cook time: 25 minutes | Servings: 6 |

Ingredients

- Shrimp - 8 oz., peeled and deveined
- Stalk lemongrass - 1, smashed
- Small ginger pieces - 2, grated
- Chicken stock - 6 cup
- Jalapenos - 2, chopped
- Lime leaves - 4
- Pineapple - 1 and 1/2 cups, chopped
- Shiitake mushroom caps - 1 cup, chopped

- Tomato - 1, chopped
- Bell pepper - 1/2, cubed
- Fish sauce - 2 tablespoons
- Sugar - 1 teaspoon
- Lime juice - 1/4 cup
- Cilantro - 1/3 cup, chopped
- Scallions - 2, sliced

Method

1. In a medium saucepan, combine ginger, lemongrass, stock, jalapenos, and lime leaves; stir, bring to a boil over medium heat, and cook for 15 minutes. Reserve the solids.

2. Return the broth to the pot, stir in the pineapple, tomato, mushrooms, bell pepper, sugar, and fish sauce, and cook for 5 minutes over medium heat. Cook for an additional 3 minutes.

3. Remove from the heat. Whisk in the lime juice, cilantro, and scallions. Ladle the soup into soup bowls and serve.

Nutritional Facts Per Serving

- Calories: 290
- Fat: 12g
- Carb: 39g
- Protein: 7g
- Sodium: 21mg

SQUID AND SHRIMP SALAD

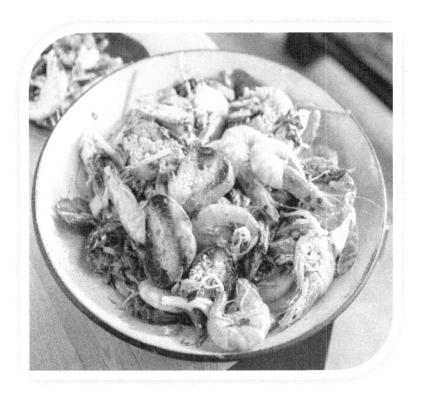

| Prep time: 10 minutes | Cook time: 15 minutes | Servings: 4 |

Ingredients

- Squid - 8 oz., cut into medium pieces
- Shrimp - 8 oz., peeled and deveined
- Red onion - 1, sliced
- Cucumber - 1, chopped
- Tomatoes - 2, cut into medium wedges
- Cilantro - 2 tablespoons, chopped

- Hot jalapeno pepper - 1, cut in rounds
- Rice vinegar - 3 tablespoons
- Dark sesame oil - 3 tablespoons
- Black pepper to the taste

Method

1. In a dish, combine the onion, cucumber, tomatoes, pepper, cilantro, shrimp, and squid. Fold a parchment paper in half, then in half-heart form.

2. Fill this parchment piece halfway with the seafood mixture, fold over, seal the edges, place on a baking sheet. Bake for 15 minutes at 400F.

3. Meanwhile, in a separate bowl, whisk together sesame oil, rice vinegar, and black pepper. Remove the salad from the oven and place it on a serving plate to cool for a few minutes before serving.

4. Drizzle with dressing and serve.

Nutritional Facts Per Serving

- Calories: 235
- Fat: 8g
- Carb: 9g
- Protein: 30g
- Sodium: 165mg

BROWN RICE CASSEROLE WITH COTTAGE CHEESE

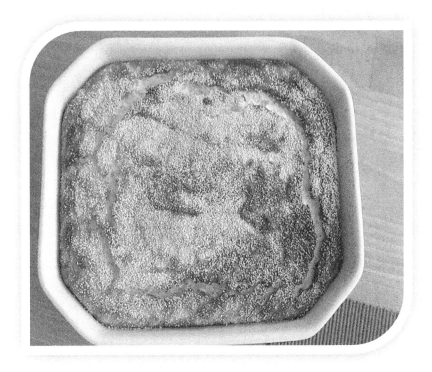

| Prep time: 15 minutes | Cook time: 45 minutes | Servings: 3 |

Ingredients

- Nonstick cooking spray
- Quick-cooking brown rice - 1 cup
- Olive oil - 1 teaspoon
- Diced sweet onion - 1/2 cup
- Fresh spinach - 1 (10-oz.) bag
- Low-fat cottage cheese - 1 1/2 cups

59

- Grated parmesan cheese - 1 tablespoon
- Sunflower seed kernels - 1/4 cup

Method

1. Preheat the oven to 375F. Spray a baking sheet with cooking spray.

2. In a casserole dish, Cook the rice according to the directions on the package. Place aside.

3. Warm the oil. Then sauté the onion for 3 to 4 minutes.

4. Cover the skillet and heat for 1 to 2 minutes, or until the spinach wilts. Remove the skillet from the heat. Combine the rice, spinach combination, and cottage cheese in a medium bowl.

5. Transfer the mixture to a casserole dish after topping with Parmesan cheese and sunflower seeds

6. Bake for 25 minutes. Serve immediately.

Nutritional Facts Per Serving

- Calories: 334
- Fat: 9g
- Carb: 47g
- Protein: 19g
- Sodium: 425mg

MOROCCAN-INSPIRED TAGINE WITH CHICKPEAS & VEGETABLES

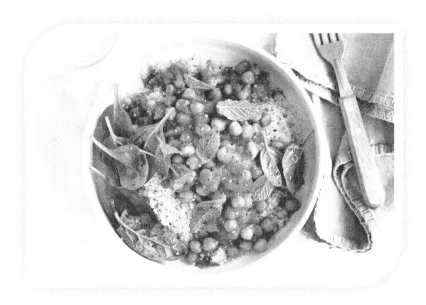

| Prep time: 15 minutes | Cook time: 45 minutes | Servings: 3 |

Ingredients

- Olive oil 2 teaspoons
- Chopped carrots 1 cup
- Finely chopped onion 1/2 cup
- Sweet potato 1, diced
- Low-sodium vegetable broth 1 cup
- Ground cinnamon 1/4 teaspoon
- Salt 1/8 teaspoon
- Chopped bell peppers 1 1/2 cups, any color

- Ripe plum tomatoes 3, chopped
- Tomato paste 1 tablespoon
- Garlic clove 1, pressed or minced
- Chickpeas 1 (15-oz.), can, drained and rinsed
- Chopped dried apricots 1/2 cup
- Curry powder 1 teaspoon
- Paprika 1/2 teaspoon
- Turmeric 1/2 teaspoon

Method

1. In a saucepan, heat oil. Cook until the carrots and onion are transparent, about 4 minutes.
2. Add sweet potato, broth, cinnamon, and salt, cook for 5 to 6 minutes.
3. Combine the peppers, tomatoes, tomato paste, and garlic in a medium bowl. Cook for 5 minutes more, stirring occasionally.
4. In the pot, combine the chickpeas, apricots, curry powder, paprika, and turmeric. Bring it to a boil. Then lower heat. Cover, and simmer for approximately 30 minutes. Serve.

Nutritional Facts Per Serving

- Calories: 469
- Fat: 9g
- Carb: 88g
- Protein: 16g
- Sodium: 256mg

BLACK BEAN BURGERS

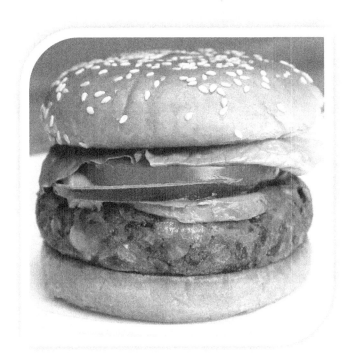

| Prep time: 15 minutes | Cook time: 20 minutes | Servings: 4 |

Ingredients

- Quick-cooking brown rice 1/2 cup (cooked according to package directions)
- Canola oil two teaspoons, divided
- Finely chopped carrots 1/2 cup
- Finely chopped onion 1/4 cup
- Black beans – 1 can, drained
- Salt-free mesquite seasoning blend 1 tablespoon
- Small hard rolls 4

Method

1. Heat 1 tsp. of oil in a skillet. Cook until the carrots and onions are transparent, about 4 minutes.

2. Reduce to low heat. Cook for another 6 minutes. Cook for 2 to 3 minutes after adding the beans and seasonings.

3. In a food processor, pulse the bean mixture three to four times or until coarsely mixed. In a bowl, blend the bean mixture and brown rice until completely incorporated. Using your hands, divide the mixture evenly and shape it into four patties.

4. In a skillet, heat the remaining oil. Cook the patties for five minutes on each side. Place the burgers on the bread and top with your favorite toppings.

Nutritional Facts Per Serving

- Calories: 368
- Fat: 6g
- Carb: 66g
- Protein: 13g
- Sodium: 322mg

LEMONGRASS AND CHICKEN SOUP

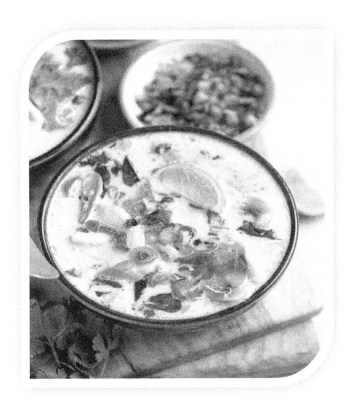

| Prep time: 10 minutes | Cook time: 25 minutes | Servings: 4 |

Ingredients

- Lime leaves - 4, torn leaves
- Veggie stock - 4 cups, low-sodium
- Lemongrass stalk - 1, chopped
- Ginger - 1 tablespoon, grated
- Chicken breast - 1-pound, skinless, boneless, and cubed
- Mushrooms 8 oz., chopped

- Thai chilies - 4, chopped
- Coconut milk - 13 oz.
- Lime juice - 1/4 cup
- Cilantro - 1/4 cup, chopped
- Pinch black pepper

Method

1. Bring the stock to a simmer in a pan. Add the lemongrass, ginger, and lime leaves and stir.
2. Cook for 10 minutes. Reheat over medium heat in another saucepan after straining. Stir in the chicken, mushrooms, milk, cilantro, black pepper, chilies, and lime juice.
3. Simmer for 15 minutes before ladling into serving bowls.

Nutritional Facts Per Serving

- Calories: 105
- Fat: 2g
- Carb: 1g
- Protein: 15g
- Sodium: 200mg

CAULIFLOWER LUNCH SALAD

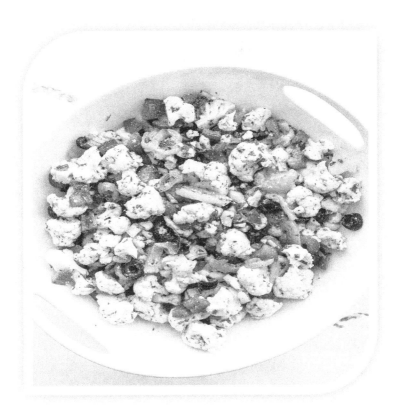

| Prep time: 120 minutes | Cook time: 10 minutes | Servings: 4 |

Ingredients

- Low-Sodium veggie stock - 1/3 cup
- Olive oil - 2 tablespoons
- Cauliflower florets - 6 cups, grated
- Black pepper to the taste
- Red onion - 1/4 cup, chopped
- Red bell pepper - 1, chopped

- Lemon juice – 1 tbsp.
- Kalamata olives halved - 1/2 cup
- Mint - 1 teaspoon, chopped
- Cilantro - 1 tablespoon, chopped

Method

1. Heat up a pan with oil. Add cauliflower, stock, and pepper. Stir and cook for 10 minutes. Transfer to a bowl and keep in the fridge for 2 hours.

2. Mix cauliflower with onion, olives, bell pepper, black pepper, mint, cilantro, lemon juice, and toss to coat.

3. Serve.

Nutritional Facts Per Serving

- Calories: 102
- Fat: 10g
- Carb: 3g
- Protein: 0g
- Sodium: 97mg

BLACK-BEAN AND VEGETABLE BURRITO

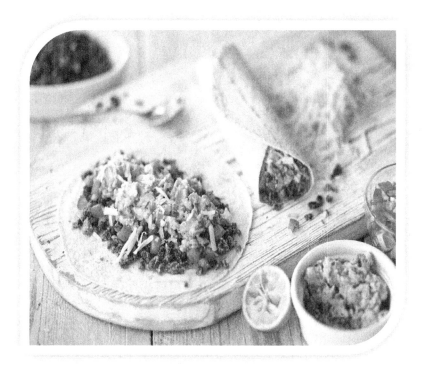

| Prep time: 15 minutes | Cook time: 15 minutes | Servings: 4 |

Ingredients

- Olive oil - 1/2 tablespoon
- Red or green bell peppers- 2, chopped
- Zucchini or summer squash - 1, diced
- Chili powder - 1/2 teaspoon
- Cumin - 1 teaspoon
- Freshly ground black pepper

- Black beans drained and rinsed - 2 cans
- Cherry tomatoes - 1 cup, halved
- Whole-wheat tortillas - 4 (8-inch)
- Optional for serving: spinach, sliced avocado, chopped scallions, or hot sauce

Method

1. In a pan, heat the oil. Sauté the bell peppers until softened, about 4 minutes.

2. Continue sautéing the zucchini, chili powder, cumin, and salt and pepper to taste until the vegetables are soft, about 5 minutes.

3. Cook for 5 minutes with the black beans and cherry tomatoes. Divide the filling among four burritos and top with your preferred toppings. Serve.

Nutritional Facts Per Serving

- Calories: 311
- Fat: 6g
- Carb: 52g
- Protein: 19g
- Sodium: 499mg

HONEY MUSTARD SALMON

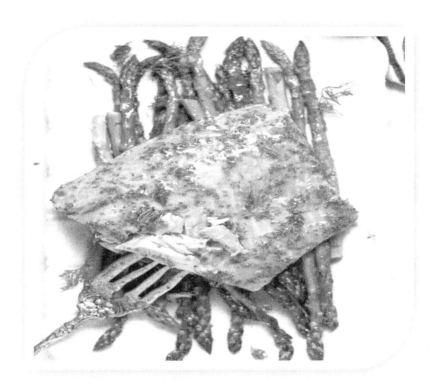

| Prep time: 5 minutes | Cook time: 15 minutes | Servings: 4 |

Ingredients

- Salmon fillets 1lb (450g) 4
- Honey mustard dressing 1 tbsp

Method

1. Preheat the oven to 400F.
2. Arrange the salmon on a sheet pan coated with parchment paper. Cook in the oven for 10 minutes.

3. Remove from the oven and spread the honey mustard dressing over the salmon.

4. Return the sheet to the oven and bake for 5 minutes more.

5. Serve.

Nutritional Facts Per Serving

- Calories: 167
- Fat: 7g
- Carb: 1g
- Protein: 23g
- Sodium: 73mg

BAKED EGGS IN AVOCADO

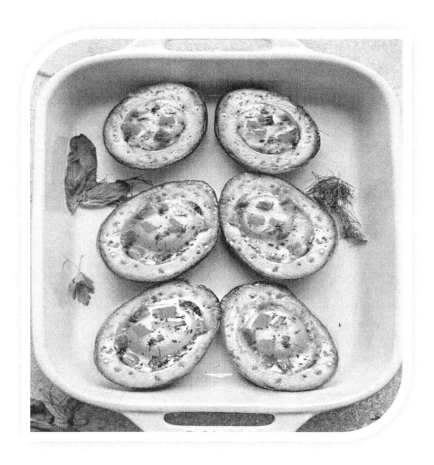

| Prep time: 15 minutes | Cook time: 15 minutes | Servings: 2 |

Ingredients

- Avocado - 2
- Limes juice - 2
- Freshly ground black pepper
- Eggs - 4

- Whole-wheat or corn tortillas - 2 (8-inch), warmed
- Optional for serving: halved cherry tomatoes and chopped cilantro

Method

1. Adjust the oven rack to the middle. Preheat the oven to 450F. Scrape out the center of halved avocado using a spoon.
2. Press lime juice over the avocados and season with black pepper to taste. Then place it on a baking sheet. Crack an egg into the avocado.
3. Bake for 10 to 15 minutes.
4. Remove from the oven. Garnish with cherry tomatoes and cilantro. Serve with warm tortillas.

Nutritional Facts Per Serving

- Calories: 534
- Fat: 39g
- Carb: 30g
- Protein: 23g
- Sodium: 462mg

Chapter 4
Dinner

CAST-IRON ROASTED CHICKEN

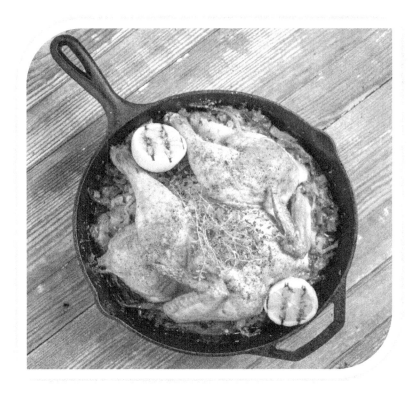

| Prep time: 20 minutes | Cook time: 80 minutes | Servings: 6 |

Ingredients

- Whole chicken - 4lb (1.8kg)
- Small bunch of fresh thyme
- Fresh rosemary - 3 sprigs
- Lemon - ½
- Garlic cloves - 3
- Olive oil - 1 tbsp

- Kosher salt - 1 tsp
- Ground black pepper

Method

1. Preheat the oven to 400F. In the center of a skillet, place the chicken. Using paper towels, pat the skin dry.
2. Insert the thyme, rosemary, lemon, and garlic into the hollow.
3. Utilize kitchen twine to secure the legs together.
4. Drizzle the olive oil over the chicken and season to taste with salt and pepper.
5. Bake for 75–80 minutes, or until the internal temperature is 165F.
6. Remove the pan from the oven carefully and set it aside to cool slightly before serving.

Nutritional Facts Per Serving

- Calorics: 293
- Fat: 10g
- Carb: 0g
- Protein: 47g
- Sodium: 153mg

LEMON & HERB GRILLED CHICKEN

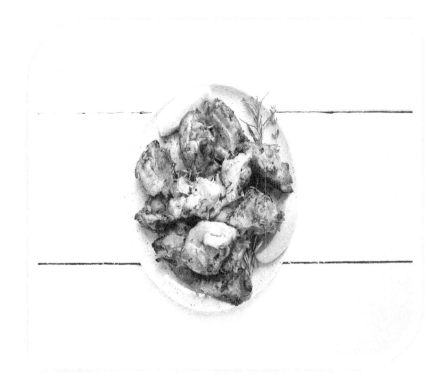

| Prep time: 10 minutes | Cook time: 15 minutes | Servings: 4 |

Ingredients

- Boneless, skinless chicken breasts - 4 (680g)
- Lemon 1, sliced
- Bunch of fresh thyme
- Fresh rosemary - 1 sprig
- Dried oregano - 1 tsp
- Honey - 2 tsp

- Balsamic vinegar - 2 tsp
- Kosher salt - 1 tsp

Method

1. Combine the chicken breasts, lemon slices, thyme, rosemary, oregano, honey, balsamic vinegar, and salt in a resealable plastic bag. Seal the bag and coat well.

2. Refrigerate the bag for a minimum of 1 hour, but up to 24 hours. Preheat the grill to medium-high. Remove the chicken from the marinade. Cook for about 6 to 8 minutes on each side, or until the inside temperature is 165F.

3. Rest and serve.

Nutritional Facts Per Serving

- Calories: 209
- Fat: 4g
- Carb: 1g
- Protein: 38g
- Sodium: 147mg

TERIYAKI CHICKEN THIGHS

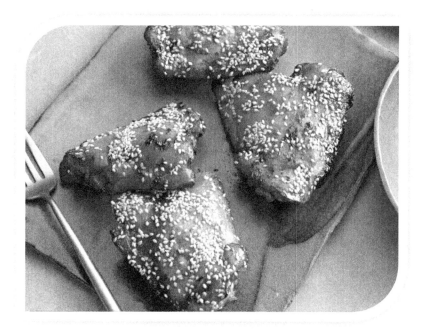

| Prep time: 5 minutes | Cook time: 20 minutes | Servings: 3 |

Ingredients

- Boneless, skinless chicken thighs 1 package (680g)
- Teriyaki sauce 3 tbsp

Method

1. Combine the chicken thighs and teriyaki sauce in a resealable plastic bag. Seal the bag coat well.

2. Refrigerate the bag on a plate or in a bowl for at least one hour but up to 24 hours. Heat the grill to medium-high. Remove the chicken and place it directly on the hot grill.

3. Cook for approximately 7 to 9 minutes per side, or until the internal temperature reaches 165F.

4. Cool and serve.

Nutritional Facts Per Serving

- Calories: 515
- Fat: 35g
- Carb: 4g
- Protein: 37g
- Sodium: 299mg

ROASTED CHILI SHRIMP

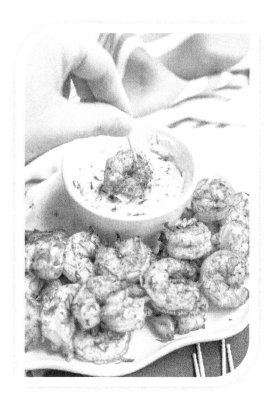

| Prep time: 5 minutes | Cook time: 10 minutes | Servings: 4 |

Ingredients

- Large shrimp 32, (450g) peeled and deveined
- Olive oil 2 tsp
- Chili powder 1 tsp
- Kosher salt ¼ tsp
- Lemon juice ½

Method

1. Preheat the oven to 425F.

2. Arrange the shrimp on a sheet pan lined with parchment paper

3. Drizzle with olive oil and season with chili powder and salt to taste.

4. Roast about 10 minutes, or until the chicken is pink.

5. Remove the baking sheet from the oven and set it aside to cool the shrimp.

6. Before serving, pour fresh lemon juice over the shrimp.

Nutritional Facts Per Serving

- Calories: 119
- Fat: 3g
- Carb: 1g
- Protein: 23g
- Sodium: 230mg

FOIL-PACKET LEMON COD

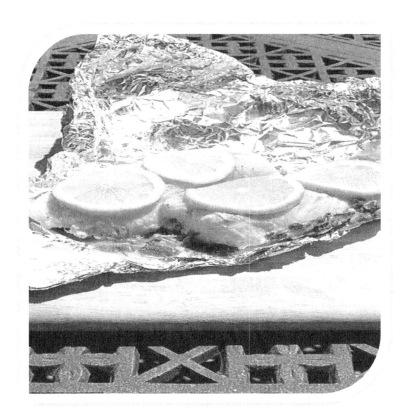

| Prep time: 5 minutes | Cook time: 10 minutes | Servings: 2 |

Ingredients

- Fresh cod fillets - 2, (225g total)
- Olive oil - 2 tbsp
- Lemon - 1, thinly sliced
- Fresh basil leaves - 1 cup
- Kosher salt - ½ tsp

- Ground black pepper - ¼ tsp

Method

1. Heat a grill to a medium-high temperature.

2. Arrange the cod fillets parallel to one another on a sheet of heavy-duty aluminum foil.

3. Each fillet should be drizzled with 1 tablespoon of olive oil, 2 lemon slices, and 1/2 cup of basil. Each fillet should be seasoned with 1 teaspoon salt and 1/8 teaspoon pepper.

4. Fold the foil's edges inward to create a packet. Place the packets on the grill and cook for approximately 10 minutes or until the salmon is opaque.

5. Using a spatula, remove the packets from the grill. Allow the fillets to cool slightly before taking them from the foil. Garnish with lemon if desired.

Nutritional Facts Per Serving

- Calories: 278
- Fat: 12g
- Carb: 0g
- Protein: 41g
- Sodium: 403mg

CHICKEN SAUSAGE PATTIES

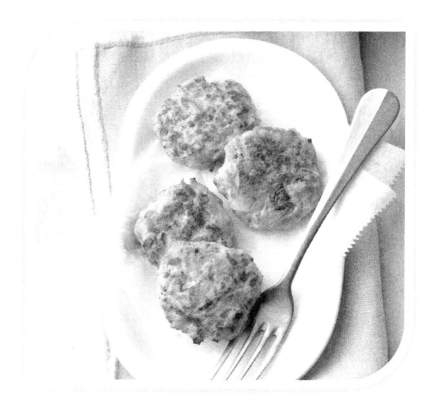

| Prep time: 10 minutes | Cook time: 20 minutes | Servings: 3 |

Ingredients

- Lean ground chicken 1lb (450g)
- Cooked brown rice ½ cup
- Chopped yellow onion ¼ cup
- Chopped garlic 2 tsp
- Ground fennel seeds 1 tsp
- Kosher salt 1 tsp

- Large egg 1, beaten

Method

1. Preheat the oven to 400F. Line a sheet pan with parchment paper.

2. Combine the ground chicken, brown rice, onion, garlic, fennel seeds, salt, and egg in a food processor. Blend until all ingredients are mixed.

3. Pour the mixture into a bowl. Shape the mixture into 9 patties with clean hands and arrange them on the prepared pan.

4. Bake until it reaches 165F, about 20 minutes. Remove the pan from the oven. Set it aside to cool the patties.

Nutritional Facts Per Serving

- Calories: 281
- Fat: 14g
- Carb: 9g
- Protein: 29g
- Sodium: 490mg

SPICY TOFU CRUMBLES

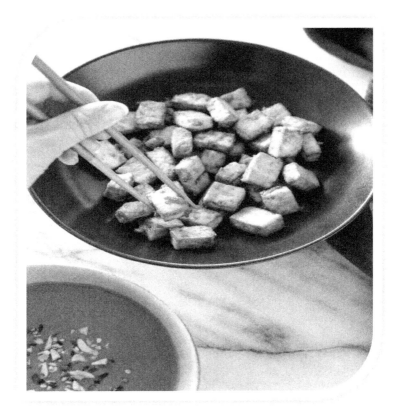

| Prep time: 5 minutes | Cook time: 20 minutes | Servings: 4 |

Ingredients

- Extra-firm tofu 1 package, drained and crumbled
- Tomato paste 2 tbsp
- Sriracha 1 tsp
- Finely chopped yellow onion ¼ cup
- Red bell pepper 1, seeded and finely chopped

- Garlic clove 1, minced
- All-purpose flour 4 tbsp
- Kosher salt ½ tsp
- Canola oil 2 tbsp

Method

1. Combine the tofu, tomato paste, sriracha, onion, bell pepper, garlic, flour, and salt in a large bowl. Combine thoroughly in a skillet heat the canola oil.

2. Sauté the tofu mixture for about 18 to 20 minutes, or until golden brown and crispy.

3. Serve.

Nutritional Facts Per Serving

- Calories: 226
- Fat: 13g
- Carb: 14g
- Protein: 13g
- Sodium: 167mg

GREEK-STYLE TURKEY BURGERS

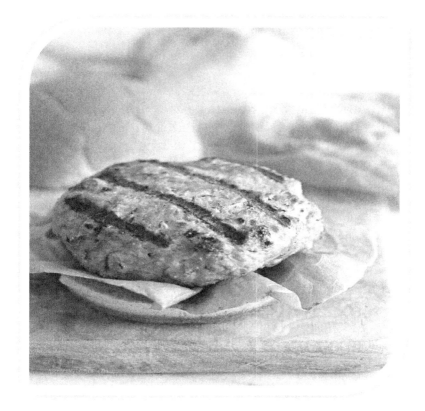

| Prep time: 10 minutes | Cook time: 16 minutes | Servings: 4 |

Ingredients

- Ground turkey breast 1lb (450g), (90% lean)
- Large egg 1, beaten
- Dried oregano 2 tsp
- Plain panko breadcrumbs ¾ cup
- Finely chopped red bell pepper ½ cup

- Kosher salt ½ tsp

Method

1. Combine the ground turkey, egg, oregano, breadcrumbs, bell pepper, and salt in a medium bowl.

2. Gently combine with clean hands and form four burgers of equal size. Heat the grill or grill pan to medium-high heat.

3. Grill the patties on the hot grill and cook for approximately 6 to 8 minutes per side, or until it reaches 165F.

4. Serve.

Nutritional Facts Per Serving

- Calories: 221
- Fat: 11g
- Carb: 7g
- Protein: 24g
- Sodium: 250mg

QUINOA & BEAN FRITTERS

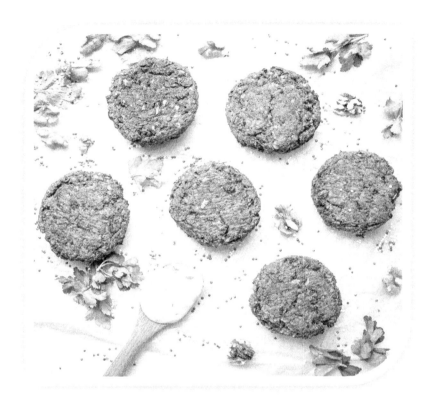

| Prep time: 10 minutes | Cook time: 25 minutes | Servings: 3 |

Ingredients

- Olive oil 1 tbsp, divided
- Small onion ½, chopped
- Kosher salt ½ tsp, divided
- Cooked quinoa 1 cup
- Chickpeas 1 can 15oz (420g), rinsed and drained
- Large egg 1

- Ground cumin ¼ tsp

Method

1. Heat 1 teaspoon of olive oil in a large skillet on the stovetop. Add the onion and 1/4 teaspoon of salt.

2. Sauté until translucent, about 4 minutes. Remove from the heat and allow the onion to cool. In a food processor, combine the onion, quinoa, chickpeas, egg, cumin, and the remaining 1 teaspoon of salt.

3. Pulse until the mixture is combined.

4. In a skillet on the stovetop, heat the remaining 2 teaspoons of olive oil over medium heat. Working in batches, place 3 spoonsful of batter in the skillet and cook for 5 to 6 minutes per side. Repeat to make 3 more fritters. Cook and serve.

Nutritional Facts Per Serving

- Calories: 248
- Fat: 9g
- Carb: 32g
- Protein: 10g
- Sodium: 377mg

LIGHTENED-UP PULLED PORK

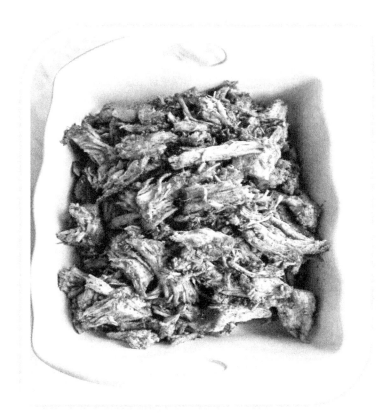

| Prep time: 10 minutes | Cook time: 60 minutes | Servings: 6 |

Ingredients

- Pork tenderloins 2, trimmed (1.4kg total)
- Apple juice ¼ cup
- Barbecue sauce ½ cup
- Ground cumin 2 tsp
- Yellow onion 1, sliced

Method

1. Cut each tenderloin into three large pieces by thinly slicing it. In a pan, combine the pork, apple juice, barbecue sauce, cumin, and onion.

2. Bring it to a boil. Then turn it down to a medium-low setting. Cook for 40 minutes, covered, rotating once or twice. Shred the pork.

3. Then, add the pork back into the stew and let it cook for another 20 minutes.

4. Remove the pot from the heat. Serve.

Nutritional Facts Per Serving

- Calories: 314
- Fat: 9g
- Carb: 8g
- Protein: 47g
- Sodium: 293mg

CRISPY SKILLET TOFU

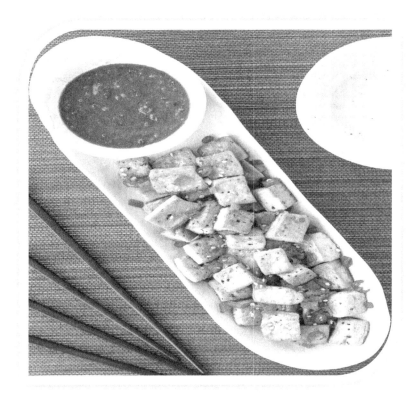

| Prep time: 10 minutes | Cook time: 20 minutes | Servings: 4 |

Ingredients

- Extra-firm tofu 1 (16oz) package, drained and cut into ½-inch cubes
- Cornstarch 1 tbsp
- Canola oil 2 tbsp
- Kosher salt ½ tsp

Method

1. To absorb excess liquid, gently press the tofu between two layers of paper towels.

2. Combine the tofu and cornstarch in a large mixing dish. To coat, toss everything together.

3. In a large nonstick skillet over medium heat, heat the canola oil. Cook, frequently rotating, until the tofu is browned and crispy on all sides, about 15 to 20 minutes.

4. Turn off the heat. Remove the skillet from the heat. Set aside to cool and season with salt. Serve.

Nutritional Facts Per Serving

- Calories: 182
- Fat: 13g
- Carb: 5g
- Protein: 11g
- Sodium: 140mg

BAKED MEATBALLS

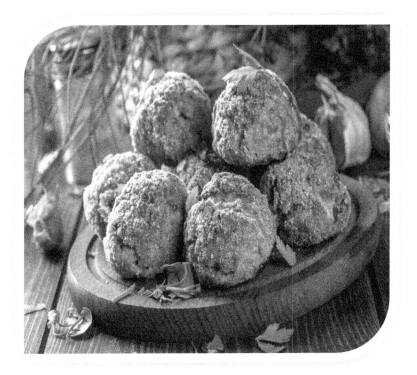

| Prep time: 10 minutes | Cook time: 20 minutes | Servings: 4 |

Ingredients

- Ground beef 1lb (450g), (90% lean)
- Large egg 1, beaten
- Panko breadcrumbs 1/3 cups
- Arugula & basil pesto 1 tbsp
- Kosher salt 1 tsp
- Ground black pepper ½ tsp

Method

1. Preheat oven to 400F.Line a sheet pan with parchment paper. In a bowl, combine the egg, ground beef, breadcrumbs, pesto, salt, and pepper.

2. Gently combine with clean hands and divide the mixture into 16 balls. Place the balls or the sheet on the table.

3. Bake for 20 minutes or until the cake reaches an internal temperature of 155F.

4. Remove the baking sheet from the oven and set it aside to cool the meatballs. Serve.

Nutritional Facts Per Serving

- Calories: 265

- Fat: 15g

- Carb: 6g

- Protein: 25g

- Sodium: 378mg

MEDITERRANEAN FLANK STEAK

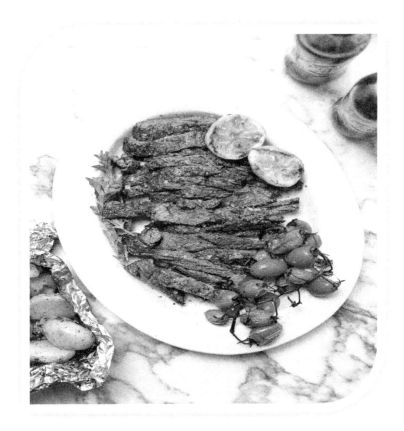

| Prep time: 10 minutes | Cook time: 16 minutes | Servings: 4 |

Ingredients

- Beef flank steak 1½lb
- Lemon juice 1 tbsp.
- Kosher salt ½ tsp
- Ground black pepper ¼ tsp
- Garlic cloves 3, minced

- Balsamic vinegar 2 tbsp
- Italian seasoning 1 tsp

Method

1. In a bowl, combine the steak, lemon juice, salt, pepper, garlic, vinegar, and Italian seasoning.
2. To coat, toss everything together. Allow at least 5 minutes, or overnight in the refrigerator, for the steak to marinade. Preheat a grill to medium-high heat.
3. Grill the steak. About 6 to 8 minutes per side, or until the desired doneness is achieved.
4. Rest, slice and serve.

Nutritional Facts Per Serving

- Calories: 241
- Fat: 9g
- Carb: 2g
- Protein: 37g
- Sodium: 233mg

DELI-STYLE TUNA SALAD

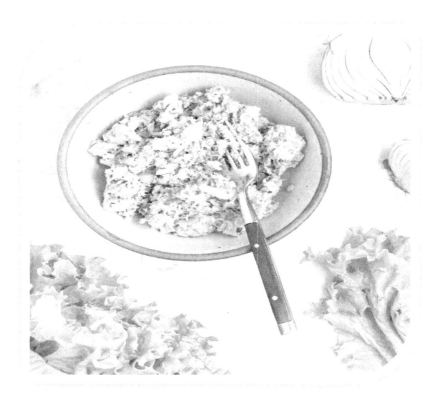

| Prep time: 10 minutes | Cook time: 10 minutes | Servings: 4 |

Ingredients

- Albacore tuna two cans (140g total), drained
- Chopped celery ½ cup
- Chopped carrot ½ cup
- Fresh parsley ½ cup
- Lemon juice 1 tbsp.
- Kosher salt ¼ tsp

- Olive oil 1 tbsp
- Mayonnaise 2 tbsp

Method

1. In a food processor, combine the olive oil, mayonnaise, salt, lemon juice, parsley, carrot, celery, and tuna. Pulse until combined.
2. Serve.

Nutritional Facts Per Serving

- Calories: 161
- Fat: 10g
- Carb: 2g
- Protein: 23g
- Sodium: 133mg

CLASSIC CHICKEN NOODLE SOUP

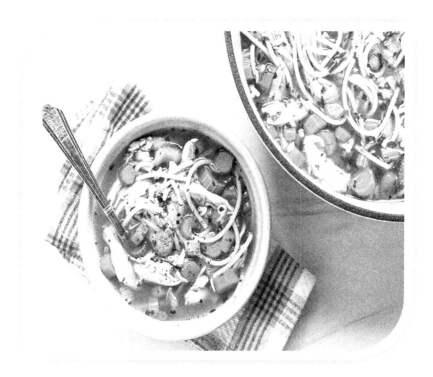

| Prep time: 10 minutes | Cook time: 20 minutes | Servings: 4 |

Ingredients

- Olive oil 1 teaspoon
- Onion 1 cup, chopped
- Cloves garlic 3, minced
- Celery 1 cup, chopped
- Carrots 1 cup, sliced & peeled
- Chicken broth 4 cups
- Linguini 4 ounces, dried & broken

- Chicken breast 1 cup, cooked & chopped
- Fresh parsley 2 tablespoons

Method

1. Heat the oil in a pan.
2. Cook until the garlic and onion are softened. Combine the celery and carrots. Cook for an additional three minutes. Then add to the broth. Bring it to a boil. Then reduce it to a simmer.
3. Cook for an additional five minutes before adding the linguine. Bring to a boil, then reduce heat.
4. Cook for an additional 10 minutes. Stir in the parsley and cook the chicken until it is thoroughly cooked.
5. Serve immediately.

Nutritional Facts Per Serving

- Calories: 381
- Fat: 12.9g
- Carb: 9.7g
- Protein: 25.3g
- Sodium: 480mg

THAI PASTA SALAD

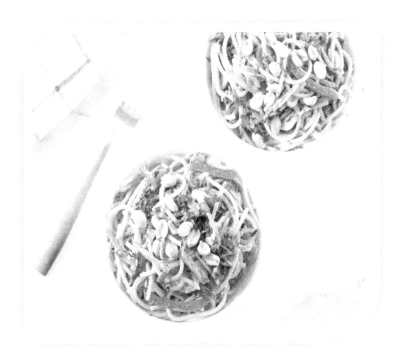

| Prep time: 15 minutes | Cook time: 14 minutes | Servings: 8 |

Ingredients

- Dry spaghetti 1 (16-oz.) package
- Peanut oil 2 tablespoons
- Medium yellow squash 1, julienned
- Medium zucchini 1, julienned
- Medium green bell pepper 1, julienned
- Red bell pepper 1, julienned
- Orange bell pepper 1, julienned
- Scallions 6, sliced
- Cloves garlic 3, minced

- Jalapeno pepper 1, minced
- Chopped walnuts 3/4 cup
- Peanut oil 1/3 cup
- Sesame oil 1 tablespoon
- Unflavored rice vinegar 1/4 cup
- Salt-free peanut butter 2 tablespoons
- No-salt-added tomato paste 1 tablespoon
- Chopped fresh cilantro 1/4 cup
- Fresh ginger 1 tablespoon, minced
- Sugar 1 teaspoon
- Salt-free chili seasoning 1/4 teaspoon

Method

1. Bring the pasta to a boil in a pot of salted water. Cook for 10 minutes, stirring once or twice during that time. Remove from the heat. Drain it, and set it aside.

2. In a large sauté pan over medium-high heat, warm 2 tablespoons of peanut oil. Cook, occasionally stirring, for 3–4 minutes before adding the julienned vegetables, scallions, garlic, jalapeno, and walnuts.

3. Remove the pan from the heat. Transfer to a bowl. Combine the cooked spaghetti with the sauce.

4. In a mixing bowl, whisk together the remaining ingredients. Drizzle over the spaghetti salad. Serve right away.

Nutritional Facts Per Serving

- Calories: 464
- Fat: 24g
- Carb: 50g
- Protein: 11g
- Sodium: 90mg

Chapter 5: Desserts

POACHED PEARS

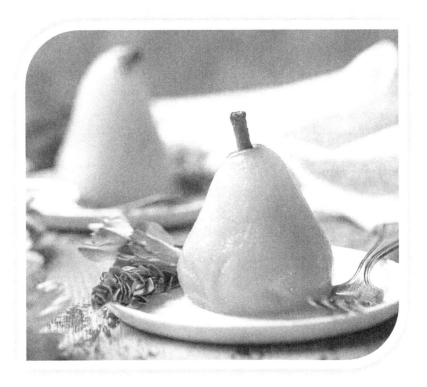

| Prep time: 15 minutes | Cook time: 30 minutes | Servings: 4 |

Ingredients

- Apple juice extract 1/4 cup
- Fresh raspberries 1/2 cup
- Orange juice extract 1 cup
- Cinnamon 1 teaspoon, ground
- Ground nutmeg 1 teaspoon
- Orange zest 2 tablespoons

- Whole pears 4, peeled, destemmed, core removed

Method

1. In a bowl, combine the cinnamon, nutmeg, fruit juices and stir.
2. In a pan, pour the juice mixture. Add the pears and turn pears frequently to maintain poaching. Do not boil. Simmer for 30 minutes.
3. Garnish with orange zest and raspberries and serve.

Nutritional Facts Per Serving

- Calories: 140
- Fat: .5g
- Carb: 34g
- Protein: 1g
- Sodium: 9mg

PUMPKIN WITH CHIA SEEDS PUDDING

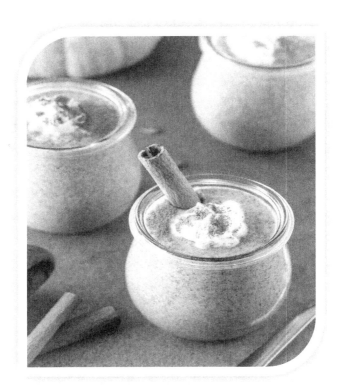

| Prep time: 60 minutes | Cook time: 65 minutes | Servings: 4 |

Ingredients

For the Pudding:

- Organic chia seeds 1/2 cup
- Raw maple syrup 1/4 cup
- Low-fat milk 1 1/4 cup
- Pumpkin puree extract 1 cup

For the Toppings:

- Organic sunflower seeds 1/4 cup
- Coarsely chopped almonds 1/4 cup
- Blueberries 1/4 cup

Method

1. Add all the ingredients for the pudding in a bowl and mix well.
2. Cover and store in a chiller for 1 hour.
3. Remove from the chiller. Transfer containers to a jar and add the ingredients for the toppings.
4. Serve.

Nutritional Facts Per Serving

- Calories: 189
- Fat: 7g
- Carb: 27g
- Protein: 5g
- Sodium: 42mg

CHOCOLATE TRUFFLES

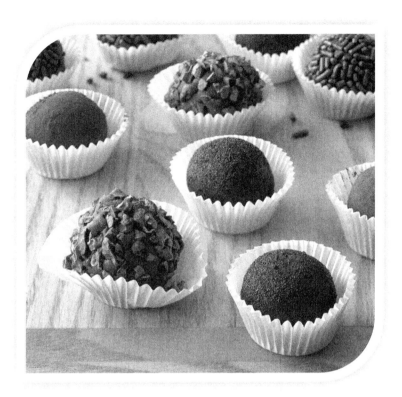

| Prep time: 15 minutes | Cook time: 10 minutes | Servings: 24 |

Ingredients

- Cacao powder 1/2 cup
- Chia seeds 1/4 cup
- Flaxseed meal 1/4 cup
- Maple syrup 1/4 cup
- Flour 1 cup
- Almond milk 2 tablespoons

For the Coatings:

- Cacao powder
- Chia seeds
- Flour
- Shredded coconut, unsweetened

Method

1. Place all the ingredients for the truffle in a blender. Blend until blended. Transfer contents to a bowl.
2. Form into chocolate balls. Then cover with the coating ingredients. Serve.

Nutritional Facts Per Serving

- Calories: 70
- Fat: 1g
- Carb: 14g
- Protein: 1g
- Sodium: 2mg

GRILLED PINEAPPLE STRIPS

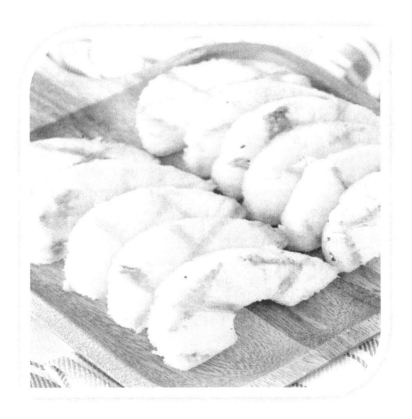

| Prep time: 15 minutes | Cook time: 5 minutes | Servings: 6 |

Ingredients

- Vegetable oil
- Pineapple 1
- Lime juice extract 1 tablespoon
- Olive oil 1 tablespoon
- Raw honey 1 tablespoon
- Brown sugar 3 tablespoons

Method

1. Remove the eyes and core from the pineapple before peeling it. Cut lengthwise to create six wedges.

2. In a bowl, whisk the remaining ingredients until smooth. Brush the pineapple with the coated mixture (reserve some for basting).

3. Vegetable oil should be used to grease an oven rack or an outside barbecue rack.

4. Arrange the pineapple wedges on the grill rack and cook for a few minutes on each side, basting regularly with the reserved glaze.

5. Arrange on a serving plate.

Nutritional Facts Per Serving

- Calories: 97
- Fat: 2g
- Carb: 20g
- Protein: 1g
- Sodium: 2mg

RASPBERRY PEACH PANCAKE

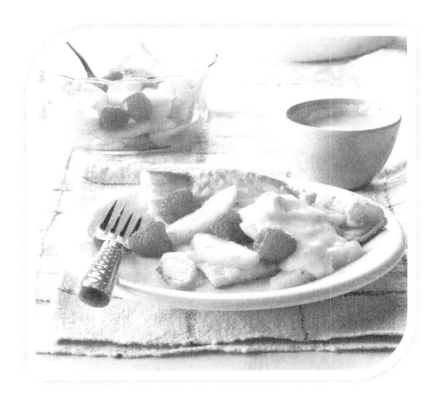

| Prep time: 15 minutes | Cook time: 30 minutes | Servings: 4 |

Ingredients

- Sugar 1/2 teaspoon
- Raspberries 1/2 cup
- Fat-free milk 1/2 cup
- All-purpose flour 1/2 cup
- Vanilla yogurt 1/4 cup
- Iodized salt 1/8 teaspoon

- Butter 1 tablespoon
- Medium peeled 2, thinly sliced peaches
- Lightly beaten organic eggs 3

Method

1. Preheat the oven to 400F. In a bowl, combine peaches and raspberries with sugar.

2. In a 9-inch circular baking dish, melt the butter. In a bowl, mix the eggs, milk, and salt until combined; whisk in the flour.

3. Remove the round baking tray from the oven and tilt it to coat the bottom and sides with melted butter. Add the flour mixture.

4. Bake it until it is browned and puffy. Take the pancake out of the oven. Serve immediately, garnished with additional raspberries and vanilla yogurt if desired.

Nutritional Facts Per Serving

- Calories: 199
- Fat: 7g
- Carb: 25g
- Protein: 9g
- Sodium: 173mg

MANGO RICE PUDDING

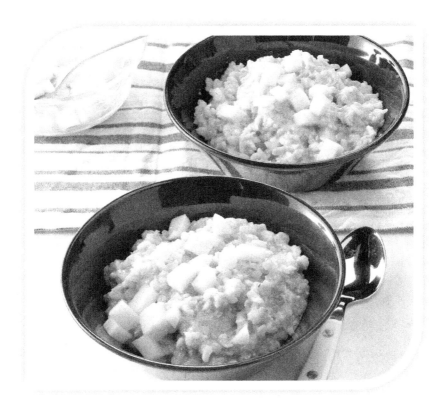

| Prep time: 15 minutes | Cook time: 35 minutes | Servings: 4 |

Ingredients

- Ground cinnamon 1/2 teaspoon
- Iodized salt 1/4 teaspoon
- Vanilla extract 1 teaspoon
- Long-grain uncooked brown rice 1 cup
- Mediums ripe mango 2, peeled, cored
- Vanilla soymilk 1 cup

- Sugar 2 tablespoons
- Water 2 cups

Method

1. To cook the rice, bring a pot of seawater to a boil; after a few minutes, reduce to low heat and cover for 30–35 minutes, or until the rice absorbs the water.

2. Using a mortar and pestle or a stainless-steel fork, mash the mango. In a saucepan, combine the rice, milk, sugar, cinnamon, and mashed mango; cook, covered, over low heat, stirring occasionally.

3. Stir in the vanilla soymilk after removing the mango rice pudding from the heat. Serve right away.

Nutritional Facts Per Serving

- Calories: 321
- Fat: 1.8g
- Carb: 71g
- Protein: 6.2g
- Sodium: 179mg

VANILLA CUPCAKES WITH CINNAMON-FUDGE FROSTING

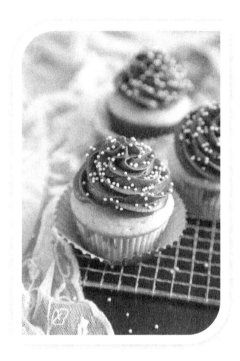

| Prep time: 10 minutes | Cook time: 18 minutes | Servings: 12 |

Ingredients

- White whole-wheat flour 1 1/2 cups
- Sugar 3/4 cup
- Sodium-free baking powder 3/4 teaspoon
- Sodium-free baking soda 1/2 teaspoon
- Nondairy milk 1 cup
- Canola oil 6 tablespoons

- Apple cider vinegar 1 tablespoon
- Pure vanilla extract 1 tablespoon

Frosting:

- Powdered sugar 2 cups
- Unsweetened cocoa powder 1/3 cup
- Non-hydrogenated vegetable shortening 4 tablespoons
- Nondairy milk 4 tablespoons
- Ground cinnamon 1 teaspoon
- Pure vanilla extract 1 teaspoon

Method

1. Preheat the oven to 350F.
2. Prepare a 12-muffin tin by lining it with paper liners and setting it aside. In a mixing dish, combine the flour, sugar, baking powder, and baking soda. Combine the remaining batter ingredients in a large mixing bowl.
3. Distribute the batter evenly among the muffin cups and bake for 18 minutes. Remove and cool on a wire rack.
4. In a mixing basin, beat the frosting ingredients until frothy. Cupcakes should be frosted. Serve right away.

Nutritional Facts Per Serving

- Calories: 347
- Fat: 7g
- Carb: 60g
- Protein: 13g
- Sodium: 46mg

CHOCOLATE CUPCAKES WITH VANILLA FROSTING

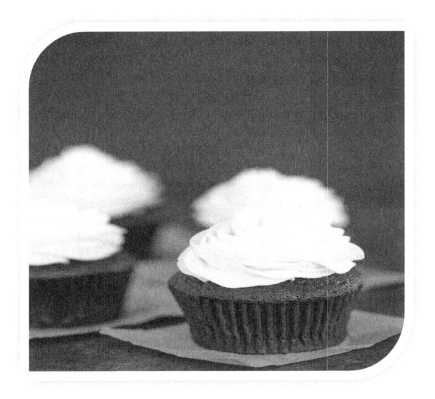

| Prep time: 15 minutes | Cook time: 20 minutes | Servings: 12 |

Ingredients

- White whole-wheat flour 1 1/2 cups
- Sugar 1 cup
- Sodium-free baking soda 2 teaspoons
- Unsweetened cocoa powder 1/4 cup
- Water 1 cup

- Canola oil 4 tablespoons
- Unsweetened applesauce 4 tablespoons
- Pure vanilla extract 1 tablespoon
- Distilled white vinegar 1 teaspoon

Frosting:

- Powdered sugar 1 1/2 cups
- Non-hydrogenated vegetable shortening 4 tablespoons
- Nondairy milk 2 1/2 tablespoons
- Pure vanilla extract 1 tablespoon

Method

1. Preheat the oven to 350F. Set aside a 12-muffin tray lined with paper liners. In a mixing dish, combine the flour, sugar, and baking soda.

2. Combine the remaining batter ingredients in a separate bowl and mix just until incorporated. Evenly distribute the batter among the muffin cups. Bake the cupcakes until a toothpick inserted in the center comes out clean, about 20 minutes.

3. Remove from the oven. Cool on a wire rack. Frost cupcakes after combining the frosting ingredients in a clean mixing bowl. Serve right away.

Nutritional Facts Per Serving

- Calories: 272
- Fat: 9g
- Carb: 45g
- Protein: 2g
- Sodium: 2mg

CHOCOLATE CHIP BANANA MUFFIN TOP COOKIES

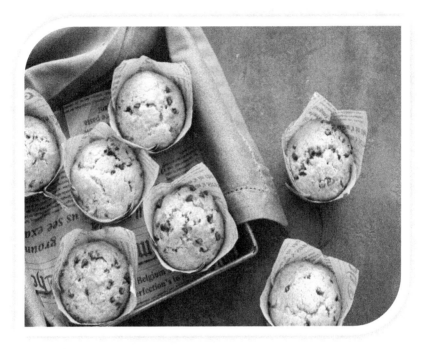

| Prep time: 15 minutes | Cook time: 15 minutes | Servings: 16 |

Ingredients

- Quick oats 1 cup
- White whole-wheat flour 1 cup
- Sugar 1/4 cup
- Sodium-free baking powder 1 tablespoon
- Ground cinnamon 1 teaspoon
- Ripe medium bananas 3, mashed

- Canola oil 4 tablespoons
- Pure vanilla extract 1 tablespoon
- Chocolate chips 3/4 cup

Method

1. Preheat the oven to 350F. Set aside a parchment-lined baking sheet. In a mixing bowl, combine the oats, flour, sugar, baking powder, and cinnamon. Add the other ingredients and mix just until incorporated.

2. Using a medium-sized ice cream scoop, scoop the batter onto the prepared baking sheet, leaving an inch or two between cookies.

3. Bake for 15 minutes. Remove from the oven and cool it on a wire rack. Serve immediately.

Nutritional Facts Per Serving

- Calories: 150
- Fat: 6g
- Carb: 23g
- Protein: 2g
- Sodium: 0mg

LEMON COOKIES

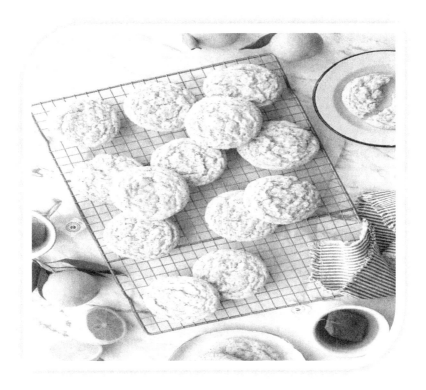

| Prep time: 15 minutes | Cook time: 10 minutes | Servings: 36 |

Ingredients

- White whole-wheat flour 2 1/2 cups
- Sugar 1 1/2 cups
- Sodium-free baking powder 1 tablespoon
- Canola oil 3/4 cup
- Large lemons 2, juice, and grated zest
- Pure vanilla extract 1 tablespoon

Method

1. Preheat the oven to 350F.

2. In a mixing dish, combine the flour, sugar, and baking powder. Combine the remaining ingredients and whisk to form a stiff dough.

3. Drop by rounded spoonfuls onto a parchment-lined baking sheet. Bake for ten minutes.

4. Remove it from the oven. Rest and serve.

Nutritional Facts Per Serving

- Calories: 106
- Fat: 5g
- Carb: 15g
- Protein: 1g
- Sodium: 0mg

PEANUT BUTTER CHOCOLATE CHIP BLONDIES

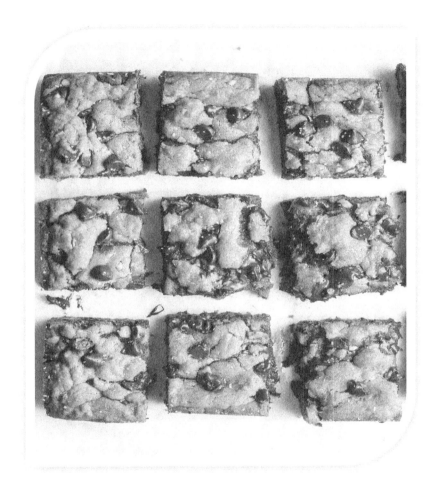

| Prep time: 15 minutes | Cook time: 20 minutes | Servings: 24 |

Ingredients

- Salt-free peanut butter 1/4 cup
- Light brown sugar 3/4 cup

- Unsweetened applesauce 1/2 cup
- Canola oil 1/4 cup
- Egg whites 2
- Pure vanilla extract 1 tablespoon
- Sodium-free baking powder 2 teaspoons
- Unbleached all-purpose flour 1 cup
- White whole-wheat flour 1/2 cup
- Semisweet chocolate chips 1/2 cup

Method

1. Preheat the oven to 400F. Set aside a 9" x 13" baking pan that has been oiled and floured. In a mixing dish, combine the peanut butter, sugar, applesauce, oil, egg whites, and vanilla extract.
2. Stir in the baking powder. Gradually incorporate the flour, stirring constantly. Incorporate the chocolate chips.
3. In the prepared pan, spread the batter evenly.
4. Bake for a total of 20 minutes. Remove and allow to cool. Cool completely before cutting into bars and serve.

Nutritional Facts Per Serving

- Calories: 18
- Fat: 5g
- Carb: 17g
- Protein: 2g
- Sodium: 7mg

GINGER SNAPS

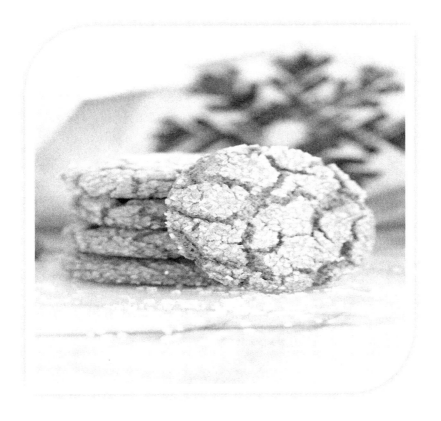

| Prep time: 15 minutes | Cook time: 10 minutes | Servings: 18 |

Ingredients

- Unsalted butter 4 tablespoons
- Light brown sugar 1/2 cup
- Molasses 2 tablespoons
- Egg white 1
- Ground ginger 2 1/2 teaspoons
- Ground allspice 1/4 teaspoon

- Sodium-free baking soda 1 teaspoon
- Unbleached all-purpose flour 1/2 cup
- White whole-wheat flour 12 cup
- Sugar 1 tablespoon

Method

1. Preheat the oven to 375F. Set aside a parchment-lined baking sheet. In a mixing bowl, combine the butter, sugar, and molasses.

2. In a mixing bowl, combine the egg white, ginger, and allspice. Combine the baking soda and baking powder, then add the flour and beat.

3. Form little balls of dough into place the balls on the prepared baking sheet and use a glass dipped in 1 tablespoon of sugar to push them down.

4. Once the glass is pressed on the dough, it will become moist enough to coat with sugar. Bake for ten minutes. Cool and serve.

Nutritional Facts Per Serving

- Calories: 81
- Fat: 2g
- Carb: 14g
- Protein: 1g
- Sodium: 6mg

CARROT CAKE COOKIES

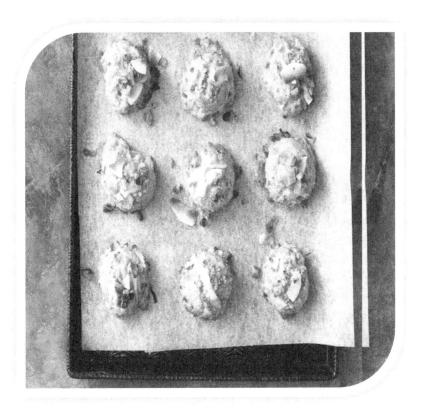

| Prep time: 15 minutes | Cook time: 12 minutes | Servings: 36 |

Ingredients

- Medium carrots 3, shredded
- White whole-wheat flour 1 1/2 cups
- Oat flour 3/4 cup
- Light brown sugar 3/4 cup
- Egg white 1
- Canola oil 1/3 cup

- Pure vanilla extract 1 tablespoon
- Sodium-free baking powder 1 teaspoon
- Ground cinnamon 1 1/2 teaspoons
- Ground nutmeg 1/2 teaspoon
- Ground ginger 1/4 teaspoon
- Ground cloves 1/8 teaspoon

Method

1. Preheat the oven to 375 Fahrenheit.
2. Arrange parchment paper on a baking pan and set it aside. Combine all the ingredients in a mixing bowl and make a dough.
3. Bake for 15 minutes on a baking sheet lined with parchment paper. Remove and cool the cookies on a wire rack.

Nutritional Facts Per Serving

- Calories: 67
- Fat: 2g
- Carb: 10g
- Protein: 1g
- Sodium: 7mg

CONCLUSION

The DASH diet has been proven to reduce the risk of heart attack, stroke, heart failure, and some cancers, including breast cancer. Additionally, the DASH diet plan lowers the risk of developing diabetes and kidney stones. The DASH diet places emphasis on consuming a variety of meals while also ensuring that the essential nutrients are being received in the optimal amounts.

Blood pressure can be lowered by eating a diet rich in fruits and vegetables. Preventing heart disease, strokes, diabetes, and weight loss are just a few of the health benefits of lowering your blood pressure. It also teaches you how to live a healthy lifestyle. This diet has received widespread praise because it adheres to guidelines already recommended by physicians. Consuming less salt, less processed meat, saturated fat, cholesterol, and trans-fat is ideal.

Printed in Great Britain
by Amazon

23158203R00079